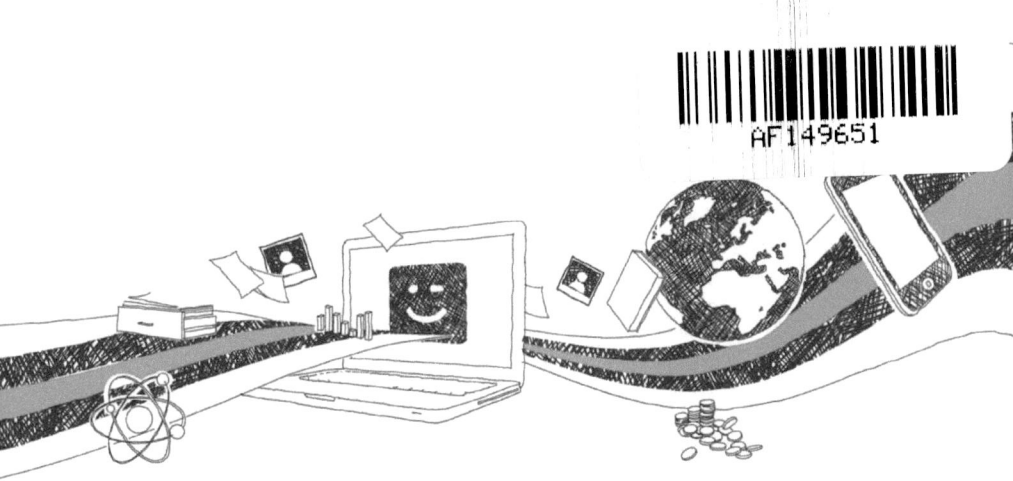
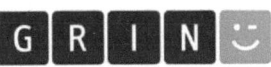

Bibliographic information published by the German National Library:

The German National Library lists this publication in the National Bibliography; detailed bibliographic data are available on the Internet at http://dnb.dnb.de .

Imprint:

Copyright © 2016 GRIN Verlag, Open Publishing GmbH
Print and binding: Books on Demand GmbH, Norderstedt Germany
ISBN: 9783668273887

This book at GRIN:

http://www.grin.com/en/e-book/337273/patient-satisfaction-with-health-care-service-providers-in-pakistan-a

Ali Adnan Joiya, Rana Saifullah Hassan, Ali Zeshan Joiya

Patient satisfaction with health care service providers in Pakistan. A review of public sector hospitals of Lahore

GRIN Publishing

GRIN - Your knowledge has value

Since its foundation in 1998, GRIN has specialized in publishing academic texts by students, college teachers and other academics as e-book and printed book. The website www.grin.com is an ideal platform for presenting term papers, final papers, scientific essays, dissertations and specialist books.

Visit us on the internet:

http://www.grin.com/

http://www.facebook.com/grincom

http://www.twitter.com/grin_com

DYNAMICS IMPACTING PATIENT SATISFACTION BY HEALTH CARE SERVICE PROVIDER. A REVIEW OF PUBLIC SECTOR HOSPITALS OF LAHORE, PAKISTAN

Ali Adnan Joiya, Rana Saifullah Hassan, Ali Zeshan Joiya

The authors of this text are not native English speakers. Please excuse any grammatical errors and other inconsistencies.

Abstract

Background:

Appropriate and improved strategies for quality assurance in the Punjab Public sector hospitals, Pakistan can be evolved with the appropriate understanding of factors influencing quality of medical service. Patient satisfaction is itself a critical controversy for the healthcare professionals/Government. Patient satisfaction is a complicated attitude because a horde of variables have been pinpointed as its interpreters. However, the study is aimed to ascertain the factors affecting the quality Healthcare services providers within Lahore Public Sector Hospitals, Punjab, Pakistan.

Objective of the Study:

The study was conducted chastely in the public interest and in order to facilitate the Govt. of Punjab, Pakistan to deal with its maximum potential to bring about ultimate satisfaction level of the patients with a foremost objective of providing fairly, attainable and effective healthcare services. The study was conducted

- To analyze factors impacting patient satisfaction in Public sector hospitals
- To rank the most important factors affecting patient satisfaction
- To evaluate the necessary steps taken by the hospital administrators for patient satisfaction.

Research Approach:

This study identified the most important factors affecting the patient satisfaction in the public sector hospitals. Surveys and interview were conducted from the 100 patients in order to come out with primary data. Further an appropriate structure questionnaire was excerpted from the available literature and expert opinion relating to the patients satisfaction from healthcare professionals. The questionnaire data was then interpreted through SPSS-20.

Conclusion:

The study ascertained the 30 most important factors resulting in poor level of patient satisfaction. Results identified that majority of the factors out of **30** factors lie in Medium and high Severity zone (with a rating between 3.4 to 4.2 out of total 5). These factors also require foremost attention by the Government. After pointing out the 30factors and their severity level, the study revealed the top 12 most important factors on the basis of Impact Factor and Relative Importance Index.

Limitations:

The study is bordered to Lahore, Punjab Public sector Hospitals, Pakistan.

Importance and Contribution:

The quality of health care services is directly linked with the satisfaction level of the patients, as the quality increase the level of patient satisfaction becomes higher. The foremost objective and purpose of this study is to facilitate the Govt., people, especially patients and healthcare service provider with plentiful information to find out the fundamentals standards of quality improvement, and to deliver a starting point for the developments in quality level that has better influence on the patient satisfaction.

KEY WORDS: Patient satisfaction and Health care institutions.

Contents

1. Introduction

Level of healthcare resources mention the healthcare quality. The foremost concern of healthcare institutions is to deliver the high quality medical facilities to all patients equally. Healthcare quality is defined as the best care received for disease; the all-inclusive it also covers the complete experience of given healthcare facilities except of errors or mistakes. Quality procedures facilitate us to differentiate the level of actual performance against benchmark. Quality shows satisfaction of patients, while satisfaction of patient's level rely on numerous factors like, food, staff behavior, techniques, strikes, diagnostic facilities, and admission procedure.

In the Eastern Mediterranean region of World Health Organization (WHO), Islamic republic of Pakistan lies it is the sixth largest nation of the world on the population basis. Within Pakistan, provision of clothing, shelter, education and Health facilities is a primary responsibility as Pakistan is a welfare state. As per Alma Ata declaration (AAD) in 1978, govt. of Pakistan was founded an wide-ranging network of basic health facilities to enhanced the convenience of the population's primary healthcare services with a main objective of delivering operative, rightfully, and available .

Healthcare services at a reasonable cost. Various reasons are impacting the patient satisfaction level and causing disappointment from the govt. provided healthcare facilities such as non-availability of staff, shortage of indispensable medicine and other equipments are major factors resulting in low satisfaction level. Although, due to various significant reasons of underutilization of health facilities provided by the Govt. hospitals, the most important aspect of patient satisfaction has not been explored to better extent in Pakistan. Patient satisfaction is not a new conception but there is no such disposition of incorporation of the patient's satisfaction delivery services as per the expectancy of patients. Hence there is no appropriate literature accessible that shows the decreased patient satisfaction with respect to govt. provided healthcare facilities across all income quintiles (from low to high socioeconomic status). Numerous studies are conducted in Pakistan regarding outpatients, indoor-patients and emergency healthcare services to determine the patient satisfaction. Various studies have been conducted in the country to explore variable level regarding patient satisfaction with the healthcare service providers.

Pakistan is a signatory of the Millennium Declaration which obligates it to achieve the Millennium Development Goals (MDGs). MDGs basically signifies a convention of the world leaders to effort in order to resolve the starvation, sickness (disease) and degradation of the environment. Health sector is one of the most significant development goal of the MDGs and three are directly related with the health sector. Numerous conducted studies shows that most of the countries will not get closer to the MDG targets without sound policy creativities. In Pakistan, primary health issues are associate with other problems. Progress of Pakistan has been impeded by the current political and economic scenario towards the MDGs that relates to health sector. Sluggish growth of economy, energy crises, humanitarian disasters, flooding, terrorism and military operations harshly   blocked the efforts made by Govt. to come out with the MDGs and it is also becoming hard to fulfill them.

The Punjab government has allocated an estimated Rs. 121.80 billion for the health budget along with an additional Rs. 2 billion so as to achieve the MDG's. Moreover, Rs 600 million have been earmarked to grant the for dialysis related facilities, Rs 8.25 billion to offer the treatment without any cost for the poor patients in public sector hospitals across the province and Rs.47.44 billion will be budgeted to be spent for the provision of advanced facilities to patients and up-gradation of healthcare institutions during current financial year. After under-standing the whole scenario, Punjab govt. has taken the inventiveness to initiate the Health Sector Reforms Program (HSRP). This inventiveness will be a stepping stone towards achiev-ing the Millennium Development Goals by 2015.

2. Review of Literature

In 2014, Mosadeghrad concluded the undeviating consequences for the providers of healthcare facilities. They are fortified to administer healthcare quality on regular basis and to also get started uninterrupted quality development programs to sustain patient satisfaction level. Conclusions are of great significance for policy makers.

Dhyana (2015) argued enlighten the significance of healthcare service provider's quality ex-tents, the study concludes with the results that" physical services" is of the foremost signifi-cance within health sector, followed by behavior of staff and admission process from patient view point. The level of understanding on healthcare quality by the experienced staff differs with most educated and highly experienced staff having "more knowledge" on healthcare quality. Quality development creativities i.e, organizational mission statement in respect of quality promise, re-engineering and reforming (redesigning) in health sector regularly, fixa-tion and implementation of bench marking within the health institution and monitoring of management to identify foremost issues relating to quality enable the healthcare authorities to provide the better quality.

Choi et al. (2005) determined with the findings that healthcare service quality is linked with patient satisfaction level, loyalty (Boshoff and Gray, 2004) and profitability and productivity of organization (Alexander et al. 2006).

5

Quality healthcare is itself a complex, subjective and multi-dimensional concept. Mosadeghrad (2013) concluded that healthcare quality is "providing the right healthcare services in a right way in the right place at the right time by the right provider to the right individual for the right price to get the right results". He ascertained a totality of 182 healthcare quality attributes comprising of 700 healthcare professionals and stakeholders including patients, executives, health providers by using the pluralistic assessment and grouped them comprising of 5 (five) categories: **environment, efficacy, effectiveness, efficiency and empathy.** Quality healthcare attributes includes such as appropriateness, competency, timeliness, reliability, privacy, affordability, continuity, equity, availability, accuracy, accessibility, acceptability, confidentiality, attentiveness, caring, responsiveness, accountability, reliability, completeness and facilities (Mosadeghrad, 2012).

As reported by Ahmad et al. (2011) Patient satisfaction is a severe issue for the providers of healthcare services. Larsson (2010) explored the basic relationship of patient satisfaction and healthcare quality awareness.

According to Chassin (2010) national accountability clearinghouse is a common place to quantity quality of health care and by using said measurements to boost the enhancement of raise transparency and health services.

Brooks-Carthonet et al. (2011) found that nurses evaluate quality measures and patient satisfaction. Mckinley (2001) has studies about factors depending on satisfaction and found Patients' relationship between received quality of healthcare services and prospect. Andaleeb et al. (2007) concluded in his study that greater the responsiveness, Assurance, and tangibility of health care providers will satisfy to patients at the greater level.

Soleimanpour et al (2011) reported that a patient Satisfaction is a major health problem now. In the Emergency department (ED), the role of gatekeeper is considered the treatment of the patient. Emergency department should have to provide quality service to attain customer's satisfaction. For monitoring and evaluating healthcare quality is fundamental (Joseph and Nichols 2007). In the competitive industry of healthcare attitude of patient and act of response is an important issue and it depends upon the hospital's brand image. Study is also suggesting that loyalty a positive hospital's brand image is depending on it brand image.

According to Hansen et al. (2008) explored that perceived quality of customer is on the development side and staff presentation of health is however hard work. According to Drapper et al. (2001) has obtained consumers views, influencing health care quality. Iliyasu et al. (2010) stated that the Surveys of total quality management have become common place in the development area.

According to Umar et al. (2011) wait to see the amount of time a patient is facing, which would affect the utilization of medical services. The performance of health care facilities can evaluate patient satisfaction. Medical facilities and hospitals to reduce waiting time administrators, human resource, logistics and other internal procedures, are needed to solve gaps, to ensure effective health care delivery system.

Norton et al. (2010) reported that internationally nurses are in short supply and local people face problem of language of nursing staff, because nurses cannot speak their language. Therefore assistance is required for translation. According to Chaker and Al-Azzab (2011) for the result of the patient satisfaction the conversation effort in the hospital should be strong and to increase satisfaction level of future. As reported by Aniza (2011) the patients' satisfaction has become increasingly important as patients with both medical cost and health services quality. Andaleeb (2000) found that customers informed healthcare selections depends upon the evaluation; it's a poor rating that hospital improves the quality of ranking. As reported by Mekoth et al. (2011) quality of service is an important element in marketing the services. Structure of the service varies from service to service standards and it is concerned with patient's satisfaction and loyalty, like, the role of procedure that produce results.

According to Rezaei et al. (2011) the effect of dose not impact on client satisfaction and client personality. Bleich et al. (2009) reported that Satisfaction of people with the health-care system, not the patient care experience, rather than depend on external factors to the health care system. Goldstein et al. (2000) reported that the Patients are satisfied with the services provider is likely to maintain loyalty. According to Lin (2009) doctors need to increase consultation with the patient.

Olivia et al. (2006) stated that food services are the most significant impact of patient satisfaction. Overtveit (1999) reported that methods and ideas to help to health care professionals and leaders working to improve system of care. (Wysong and Driver 2011).

3. Methodology

The present survey was a descriptive study, aimed to collect data regarding patient satisfaction in the Public health sector Punjab, Pakistan. The methodology is described as follow

1. **Selection of Factors:**

    Factors affecting were selected on the basis of a thorough literature review and expert opinions, numerous factors affecting patient satisfaction were identified in the Public health sector Punjab, Pakistan scenario. A totality of thirty (30) factors(Table 1) were selected to form survey questionnaire.

2. **Research Design:** Research design adopted was quantitative research approach in which Quantitative surveys are designed to obtain information (Rossi et al. 1983). In such surveys, information level about the population gathered through sampling method (Rea and Parker 2012). Data was clustered using Survey (Ramboll 2014).

3. **Data Collection:** The approach for data collection was primarily and it was done through field survey.

4. **Structure of Questionnaire:** Questionnaire was divided into two parts A and B. Part A was comprising of personal information like Age, Organization, Salary Range, Contact #, Gender and Address. Part B was designed to acquire the relevant information regarding patient satisfaction.

5. **Sample Size:** Survey was drained with the help of personal interviews, questionnaires were filled according to the likert scale. Respondents filled the survey as per their feelings and experience got during their treatment. One hundred (100) patients of Public sector hospitals in Lahore were approached for these surveys out of which 90 respondents filled the questionnaire sues fully.

6. **Identification of Factors:** Factors affecting patient satisfaction were pointed out in the light of literature review and expert opinions from the healthcare professionals. In this study literature review from both developed and developing countries has been studied. The finalized factors affecting patient satisfaction are shown below in Table 1. A totality of 30 factors is selected in order to come out with this study.

Table 1: Factors affecting patient satisfaction

Sr.#	Factor ID	Factor
1	PSF1	Frequent Paramedical Strikes
2	PSF2	Food
3	PSF3	In-sufficient/In-efficient Emergency Services
4	PSF4	User Friendly Systems
5	PSF5	Relevant Staff availability
6	PSF6	Prejudice dispersal of Locally purchased medicine
7	PSF7	Response to complaints
8	PSF8	Behavior of Staff
9	PSF9	Procedural information
10	PSF10	Slow/Length of Treatment
11	PSF11	Political Influence
12	PSF12	Protocols
13	PSF13	Online patient facilitation system

8

14	PSF14	Discrimination in Health facilities to patients
15	PSF15	Monitoring by Govt.
16	PSF16	Developmental Projects
17	PSF17	Surprise visits by Management
18	PSF18	Diagnostic Services
19	PSF19	Role of Management in problem identification
20	PSF20	Staff Competency
21	PSF21	Response time to a patient
22	PSF22	Inappropriate departmental Communication
23	PSF23	Staff motivation and satisfaction
24	PSF24	Non-availability of Free medicine
25	PSF25	Organizational Structure
26	PSF26	Poor Patient Care
27	PSF27	Cleanliness
28	PSF28	Admission Procedure
29	PSF29	Experienced Staff
30	PSF30	Briberies/Corruption

7. **Relative Importance Index:** It is used to indicate the relative importance of variables resulting poor quality of the healthcare institutions and it was calculated with the formula below:

$$\text{RII} = \frac{\sum W}{A \times N}$$

Where:

RII - Relative Importance Index,

W = weighting given to each factor by the respondents (ranging from 1 to 5)

A = highest weight (i.e. 5)

N = total number of respondents.

8. **Impact of 30 Factors:** Impact of each factor used to calculate the impact of each factor on the variable that is quality provided by healthcare institutions and factors are the attributes of patient satisfaction level.

$$\textbf{\textit{Impact}} = \frac{\sum (f_i \times i)}{n}$$

Where:

i = is the severity score from 1 to 5

f_i = is the frequency of factor getting score i

n = number of responses

4. Data Presentation and Analysis

As stated before, the study is conducted on the quantitative basis which demands that data should be hypothetically checked on the **SPSS-20.**

As indicated in table below, thirty (30) factors affecting the satisfaction level of the patients from the healthcare institutions in the Punjab were identified and ranked. The **30**factors that are affecting the patient satisfaction as stated above. Out of circulated 100 questionnaires only 90 were completed thoroughly. Below table is showing the results from RII and Impact of the 30 factors in order to rank and prioritize the said factors.

Table 2: RII and Impact Results

Sr .#	Factor ID	Factor	Total (n)	Weight ($\sum w$)	A	Impact	RII	Rank
1	PSF1	Frequent Paramedical Strikes	90	268	5	4.123	0.825	2nd
2	PSF2	Food	90	232	5	3.569	0.714	21st
3	PSF3	In-sufficient/In-efficient Emergency Services	90	262	5	4.031	0.806	5th
4	PSF4	User Friendly Systems	90	237	5	3.646	0.729	19th
5	PSF5	Relevant Staff availability	90	220	5	3.385	0.677	24th
6	PSF6	Prejudice dispersal of Locally purchased medicine	90	260	5	4.000	0.800	7th
7	PSF7	Response to complaints	90	211	5	3.246	0.649	27th
8	PSF8	Behavior of Staff	90	270	5	4.154	**0.831**	1st
9	PSF9	Procedural information	90	250	5	3.846	0.769	15th
10	PSF10	Slow/Length of Treatment	90	253	5	3.892	0.778	10th
11	PSF11	Political Influence	90	254	5	3.908	0.782	9th
12	PSF12	Protocols	90	249	5	3.831	0.766	16th
13	PSF13	Online patient facilitation system	90	248	5	3.815	0.763	17th
14	PSF14	Discrimination in Health facilities to patients	90	248	5	3.815	0.763	18th
15	PSF15	Monitoring by Govt.	90	251	5	3.862	0.772	13th
16	PSF16	Developmental Projects	90	219	5	3.480	0.674	22nd
17	PSF17	Surprise visits by Management	90	225	5	3.462	0.692	23rd
18	PSF18	Diagnostic Services	90	262	5	4.031	0.806	6th
19	PSF19	Role of Management in problem identification	90	251	5	3.862	0.772	14th
20	PSF20	Staff Competency	90	235	5	3.615	0.723	28th

10

21	PSF21	Response time to a patient	90	264	5	4.062	0.812	4th
22	PSF22	Inappropriate departmental Communication	90	252	5	3.877	0.775	12th
23	PSF23	Staff motivation and satisfaction	90	216	5	3.323	0.665	25th
24	PSF24	Non-availability of Free medicine	90	265	5	4.077	0.815	3rd
25	PSF25	Organizational Structure	90	236	5	3.631	0.726	20th
26	PSF26	Poor Patient Care	90	253	5	3.892	0.778	11th
27	PSF27	Cleanliness	90	256	5	3.938	0.788	8th
28	PSF28	Admission Procedure	90	211	5	3.246	0.649	29th
29	PSF29	Experienced Staff	90	207	5	3.185	0.637	30th
30	PSF30	Briberies/Corruption	90	213	5	3.277	0.655	26th

Figure 1Impact range of Factors

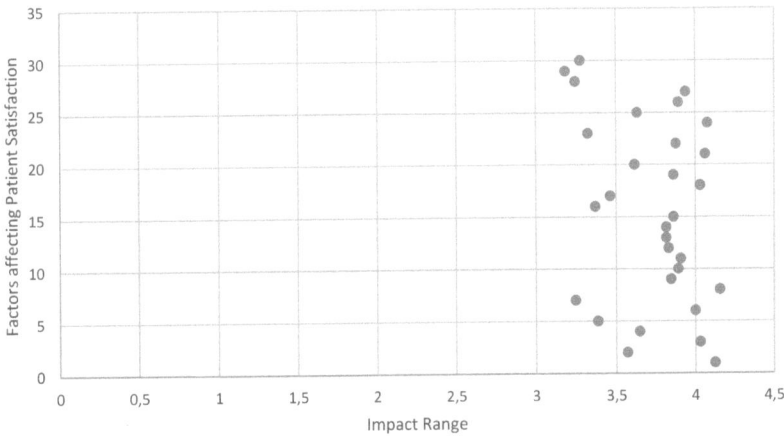

Figure 1 shows the impact range of the 30 factors impacting patient satisfaction as depicted by the data. Impact range has been divided into three clusters as described below

Low Severity Range: 1.25 to 2.5 (Impact Score)

Medium Severity Range: 2.5 to 3.75 (Impact Score)

High Severity Range: 3.75 to 5 (Impact Score)

Results shows that Results represents that all the factors lies in the medium and high severity ranges. Majority of the factors lies in the high severity range which shoes that most of the factors have high severity while impacting the patient satisfaction.

Relative Importance Index:

Relative importance index showing the significance of each factors and it also shows the ranking of factors resulting in poor quality within Lahore healthcare institutions, Punjab, Pakistan. The factors which are affecting the quality of healthcare institutions are mentioned at Table#2. Table illustrates the top 12 significant factors resulting in poor level of satisfaction level and eminence of Healthcare system as well. The most important factors according to the acuity of patients are: **"Behavior of Staff" as the 1st most important factor** that is affecting the satisfaction level at its full strength and its RII came to **"0.831"**.Similarly 12 factors were ranked according to their RII value shown in Table 3.

Table 3: Top 12 Ranked Factors According to RII values

Sr.#	Factor ID	Factor affecting Patient Satisfaction	RII	Rank
1	PSF8	Behavior of Staff	0.831	1st
2	PSF1	Frequent Paramedical Strikes	0.825	2nd
3	PSF24	Non-availability of Free medicine	0.815	3rd
4	PSF21	Response time to a patient	0.812	4th
5	PSF3	In-sufficient/In-efficient Emergency Services	0.806	5th
6	PSF18	Diagnostic Services	0.806	6th
7	PSF6	Prejudice dispersal of Locally purchased medicine	0.800	7th
8	PSF27	Cleanliness	0.788	8th
9	PSF11	Political Influence	0.782	9th
10	PSF10	Slow/Lengthy Treatment	0.778	10th
11	PSF26	Poor Patient Care	0.778	11th
12	PSF22	Inappropriate Departmental Communication	0.775	12th

Impact of Factor:

It was calculated to show the impact of each satisfaction level on the quality of healthcare institutions. Out of the 30 most common and foremost factors, 12 factors were ranked and their impact is calculated as shown in the table # 4. It is concluded that the impact factor of "Behavior of Staff" came to 4.154 at scored the highest position it also ranked as 1st. It also means that most impacting factor is Behavior of Staff. Similarly the other factors are also impacting accordingly as shown in Table 4.

Table 4: Top 12 Ranked Factors According to Impact values

Sr.#	Factor ID	Factor affecting Patient Satisfaction	Impact	Rank
1	PSF8	Behavior of Staff	4.154	1st
2	PSF1	Frequent Paramedical Strikes	4.123	2nd
3	PSF24	Non-availability of Free medicine	4.077	3rd
4	PSF21	Response time to a patient	4.062	4th
5	PSF3	In-sufficient/In-efficient Emergency Services	4.031	5th
6	PSF18	Diagnostic Services	4.031	6th
7	PSF6	Prejudice dispersal of Locally purchased medicine	4.000	7th
8	PSF27	Cleanliness	3.938	8th
9	PSF11	Political Influence	3.908	9th
10	PSF10	Slow/Lengthy Treatment	3.892	10th
11	PSF26	Poor Patient Care	3.892	11th
12	PSF22	Inappropriate Departmental Communication	3.877	12th

5. Conclusion

The primary objective of healthcare institutions is to revamp the quality level and health status of the population. The stakeholders in healthcare institutions are too vigilant about the reforms in the health sector worldwide with the aim to develop maximum level of patient satisfaction from healthcare service. Patient satisfaction is only the key marker to label the quality of health sector and represents this internationally accepted factor needs to be greatly observed for smooth functioning of the healthcare systems. Patient is the best judge since he/she accurately assesses and his /her inputs help in the overall improvement of quality health care provision through the rectification of the system weaknesses by the concerned authorities. The quality of health care services is directly linked with the satisfaction level of the patients, as the quality increase the level of patient satisfaction becomes higher.

The results of this research will allow a better understanding of the facilitators and barriers of quality medical services. The results will also enhance our understanding of the determinants of the factors influence quality of medicals services. It is anticipated that a better understanding of these factors and their relationships can pinpoint better strategies for quality assurance in medical services, particularly in Pakistan but probably in other societies as well.

- The results shows that widely held factors fall in the medium severity impact range. Significant consideration should be given to those factors.
- This study however subsidizes the foremost and leading factors patient satisfaction and ultimately poor quality system of health care institutions.

13

- This study further also prioritized the top twelve most vital factors out of thirty affecting patient satisfaction within Lahore, Punjab, Pakistan on the basis of severity impact score received.
- This study also enable the Govt., people, especially patients and healthcare service provider with plentiful information to find out the fundamentals standards of quality improvement, and to deliver a starting point for the developments in quality level that has better influence on the patient satisfaction.

6. Recommendation

The elementary purpose of this study was to develop the understanding with the factors that resultantly stand against the poor satisfaction level of the patients. Necessary measures should be adopted in the light of given ranking and the said factors may be taken on high priority just to resolve them. The most important and high priority factors should be taken to ending. Patient dealing trainings should be given to the staff that will enable them to understand the patient demands and that will remove the most impacting factor of patient satisfaction that is **"Behavior of Staff"**. Management should also take a part in the monitoring wing and special attention could be given to the complaints of the patient that makes the patients more confident.

7. REFERENCES

Andaleeb, S.S, N. Siddiqui., and S. Khandakar.2007. Patient satisfaction with health services in Bangladesh. Health Policy and Planning 2007 Jul; 22(4):263-73.

Andaleeb, S.S. 2000. Public and private hospitals in Bangladesh: service quality and Predictors of hospital choice. Health policy and planning, 15(1):95–102.

Ahmad I., A. Nawaz and S. Uddin. 2011. Dynamics of patient satisfaction from health care services.*Gomel Journal of Medical Sciences*, 9(1):37-41.

Ali Muhammad (2014), Factors Affecting Medical Service Quality, *Iranian J Publ Health, Vol. 43, No.2, Feb 2014, pp.210-220.*

Alexander JA, Weiner BJ, Griffith J (2006). Qualityimprovement and hospital financial performance.Journal of Organisational Behaviour, 27 (7): 1003-1029.

Aniza, I, M. Rizal., M. Mardhiyyah., I. Helmi, B. Syamimi, and M. Tahar. 2011. Caregivers' Satisfaction of Healthcare Delivery at Pediatric Clinics of UniversityKebangsaan Malaysia Medical Centre in 2009. *Medical Journal of Malaysia*, 66(2):84-8.

Bleich, S.N., E. Özaltin. And C. Murray. 2009. How does satisfaction with the health-caresystemrelate to patient experience? Bulletin of the World Health Organization, 87(4):271-278.

Boshoff C, Gray B (2004). The relationships between service quality, customer satisfactionand buying intentions in the private hospitalindustry. *South African Journal of Business Management*, 35 (4): 27-37.

Brooks-Carthon J.M., A. Kutney-Lee., S, D. M. Ioane., J. P. Cimiotti., L. H. Aiken. 2011. Quality of Care and Patient Satisfaction in Hospitals with High Concentrations of Black Patients. *Journal of Nursing Scholarship*, 43(3):301–310.

Chassin, M. R., J. M. Loeb, S. P. Schmaltz, R. M. Wachter. 2010. New England journal of medicine.Accountability Measures Using Measurement to Promote Quality Improvement.*AORN Journal*,363(7):683-688.

Chakraborty, R, and A. Majumdar.2011. Measuring consumer satisfaction in health care Sector: the applicability of servqual. Journal of arts, science & commerce.*International Refereed Research Journal*, 2(4):149-60.

Chaker, M, and N. Al-Azzab.2011. Patient Satisfaction in Qatar Orthopedic and Sports Medicine Hospital (ASPITAR). *International Journal of Business and Social Sciences*, 2(7):69-78.

Choi K, Lee H, Kim C, Lee S (2005). The servicequality dimensions and patient satisfaction relationshipsinSouthKorea:comparisons acrossgender, age and types of service. *Journal of ServicesMarketing*,19(3):140-9.

Drapper, M, N. Bushan. and P. Cohen. 2001. Seeking consumer view: what use are results of hospital patient satisfaction surveys. *International Journal for Quality in Health Care*, 13(6):463-468.

Goldstein, M.S, S. Elliott., and A. Guccione.2000. The Development of an Instrument to Measure Satisfaction with Physical Therapy. Physical Therapy, 80(9):853-63.

Hansen, P. M., D. H. Peters, K. Viswanathan, K. D. Rao, A. Mashkoor, G. Burnham. 2008. Client perceptions of the quality of primary care services in Afghanistan. *International Journal for Quality inHealth Care*, 20(6):384–391.

Iliyasu, Z. S. Abubakar., S. Abubakar., S. Lawan, A. Gajida. 2010. Patients' Satisfaction with Services Obtained from Aminu Kano Teaching Hospital, Kano, and Northern Nigeria. *Nigerian Journal of Clinical Practices*, 13(4):371-378.

Joseph, I, C. and S. Nichols. 2007. Patient Satisfaction and Quality of Life among Persons Attending Chronic Disease Clinics in South Trinidad, West Indies. *West Indian Medical Journal*, 56(2):108-14.

16

Larsson, G. 2010. Quality of Care and Patient Satisfaction: A New Theoretical and Methodo-logicalApproach. *International Journal of Health Care Quality Assurance*, 23(2):228-247.

Lin, D. J. 2009. Measuring Patient's Expectation and the Perception of Quality in LASIK Ser-vices. Health and Quality of Life Outcomes, 7(63).

Mekoth, N, G. Babu, Y. Dalvi, N. Rajanala, K. Nizomadinov. 2011. Service Encounter Relat-ed Process Quality, Patient Satisfaction, and Behavioral Intention. Management, 6(4):333-350.

Mosadeghrad AM, Ferlie E, Rosenberg D (2011).A Study of relationship between job stress,quality of working life and turnover intentionamong hospital employees. *Health Services ManagementResearchJournal*,24(4):170-181.

Mosadeghrad AM (2012). A Conceptual frameworkfor quality of care. *Mat Soc Med.* 24(4):251-261.

Mosadeghrad AM (2013). Healthcare service quality:Towards a broad definition. *Internation-al Journal of Health Care Quality Assurance*, 26 (3):203-219.

McKinley, R. K. 2001. Patient Satisfaction with out of Hour's Primary Medical Care. *Journal QualityHealth Care.*10(1):23-82.

Norton. D, S. Robertson, R. Anderson. 2010. A Randomized Controlled Trial to Assess the Impact of an Admission Service on Patient and Staff Satisfaction. *International Journal of Nursing Practice*, 16(5):461-471.

Olivia R. L, B. Connely, S. Capra. 2006. Consumer Evaluation of Hospital Foodservice Qual-ity:Empirical Investigation. *International Journal of Health Care Quality Assurance*, 19(2):181-194.

Rezaei. M, H. Rezaei, H. Alipour, S. Salehi. 2011. Service Quality, Client Satisfaction and Client Personality in the Public Companies. *Australian Journal of Basic and Applied Sciences*, 5(3):483-491.

Soleimanpour, H. C. Gholipouri, S. Salarilak, P. Raoufi, R. G. Vahidi, A. J. Rouhi, R. R. Ghafouri and M.Soleimanpour. 2011. Emergency Department Patient Satisfaction Survey in Imam Reza Hospital, Tabriz, Iran. *International Journal of Emergency Medicine*, 4(2).

Umar I., M. O. Oche, and A. S. Umar. 2011. Patient Waiting Time in a Tertiary Health Institution in Northern Nigeria. *Journal of Public Health and Epidemiology*, 3(2):78-82.

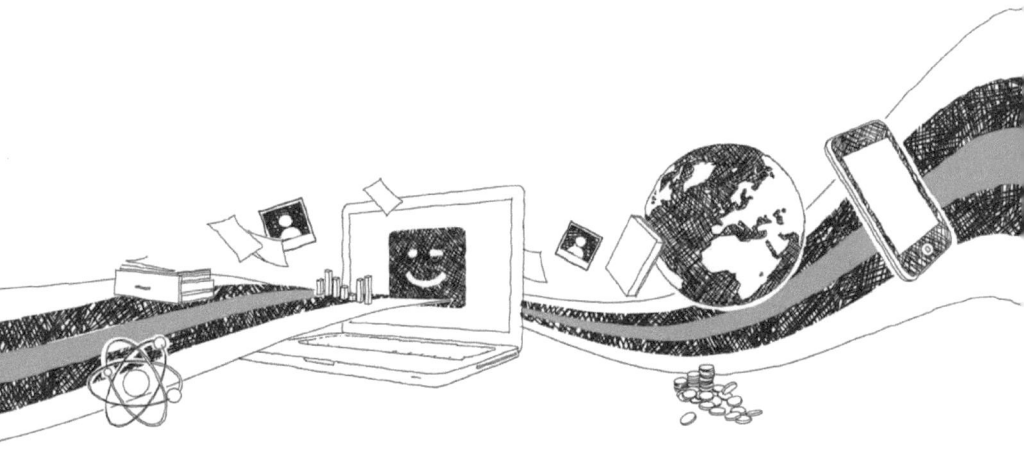
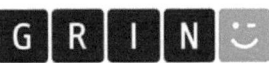